THE GOLDEN HOUR:

Nurturing Birth, Overcoming Interventions, and Establishing a Successful Breastfeeding Journey

Elisha Anderson

Copyright © 2023 Elisha Anderson

All rights reserved.

DEDICATION

To my dearest clients, both past and present, and to the mothers I will have the privilege to support in the future,

Your courage, strength, and unwavering dedication to breastfeeding have inspired me beyond measure. Each of you has illuminated my path with your unique stories, teaching me the true essence of resilience and love. It is your trust and faith in the breastfeeding journey that has fueled the pages of this book.

May these words serve as a guiding light, offering you knowledge, reassurance, and the unwavering belief in your own innate abilities. With every latch, every drop of nourishment, and every tender moment shared, you are creating a legacy of love and connection.

In deepest gratitude for allowing me into your lives and hearts, and for reminding me daily of the extraordinary strength within every mother.

With boundless love,

Elisha Anderson

CONTENTS

1	Golden Hour	1
2	Natures Perfect Beginning	5
3	Nurturing the First Latch	12
4	Herbal Remedies for Breastfeeding Complications	20
5	PUMPING	28
6	Weaning With Love	31
7	Sanctuary of Support	41

CHAPTER 1
The Golden Hour

In the hush of the birthing room, where life takes its first breaths and love expands to encompass a new soul, there exists a sacred period, a fleeting moment that holds immeasurable power – the Golden Hour. As a doula who has stood witness to countless births and as a mother who has cradled two babies at my breast, I understand the profound significance of this hour.

My book, "The Golden Hour: Nurturing Birth, Overcoming Interventions, and Cultivating a Joyful Breastfeeding Journey," is more than just a guide. It's a tapestry woven with threads of natural wisdom, compassionate advocacy, and the resilient spirit of mothers. Within these pages, we embark on a transformative journey, celebrating the innate ability of women to birth and breastfeed with confidence, even in the face of societal pressures and medical interventions.

In the heart of this book lies my own story, a narrative shaped by years of supporting mothers through the delicate dance of birth and breastfeeding. It's a tale of perseverance, of advocating for the rights of mothers to experience the Golden Hour, undisturbed and connected with their newborns. With each passing year of my own breastfeeding journey, I have seen the transformative impact of embracing this sacred hour – a time when oxytocin flows, when the first latch occurs, and when the foundation for a profound breastfeeding relationship is laid.

As we dive into the depths of this book, we will explore the natural rhythms of childbirth, the interventions that may arise, and the tender art of breastfeeding. We will unravel the healing power of herbal remedies, providing holistic solutions for common breastfeeding challenges. Together, we will navigate the realm of pumping, ensuring that every drop of mother's milk is cherished, regardless of the vessel that carries it to the baby's lips.

But this book is not just about practical advice; it's about honoring the emotional journey of motherhood. It's about validating the fears, the triumphs, and the silent battles that every mother faces. It's a testament to the strength of mothers, the resilience of newborns, and the enduring power of the Golden Hour to shape the course of a breastfeeding relationship.

In the chapters that follow, you will find stories of triumph, herbal remedies that nurture both body and soul, and guidance on how to navigate the complexities of birth interventions with grace and confidence. My hope is that within these pages, you find not just information, but a source of comfort, inspiration, and unwavering support. Together, let's embrace the Golden Hour, for within its gentle embrace lies the key to a joyful, connected, and empowering breastfeeding journey.

CHAPTER 2:
Natures Perfect Beginning

In the quiet moments after birth, when the world holds its breath and time seems to stand still, a remarkable transformation unfolds – the Golden Hour. It is within this sacred span of time that the purest essence of motherhood and the primal instincts of a newborn converge, creating a symphony of love, warmth, and connection. In this chapter, we explore the awe-inspiring wonder of the Golden Hour, delving into its physiological and emotional significance, and understanding how it lays the foundation for a harmonious breastfeeding relationship.

I. The Physiology of Skin-to-Skin Contact

A. Oxytocin: The Hormone of Love and Bonding

In the tender moments following birth, the hormone oxytocin surges through both mother and baby, weaving an unbreakable bond. Often referred to as the "love hormone" or "bonding hormone," oxytocin plays a central role in orchestrating the magical connection that occurs during the Golden Hour. This hormone not only fosters emotional intimacy but also triggers the milk ejection reflex, essential for breastfeeding.

The gentle touch, the scent, and the warmth of the mother's skin stimulate the release of oxytocin, fostering a sense of security and love for the newborn. As the baby nestles close, skin-to-skin, the mother's body responds with a surge of this powerful hormone, deepening the connection and encouraging the baby to latch onto the breast.

B. Temperature Regulation and Stability

Skin-to-skin contact acts as a natural thermostat, regulating the baby's body temperature with incredible efficiency. The mother's chest provides the perfect microclimate, adjusting to the baby's needs. For a newborn, maintaining a stable body temperature is crucial, and the comforting warmth of the mother's body ensures the baby feels safe and secure, allowing them to focus on breastfeeding.

C. Natural Instincts: Rooting and First Latch

Babies are born with an innate ability to seek out the nourishment they need. This instinct is beautifully showcased through the rooting reflex, a baby's natural instinct to turn their head and open their mouth when their cheek is gently stroked. Guided by this instinct, the baby finds the mother's breast and begins the intricate dance of latching on.

In the Golden Hour, the first latch is more than a mere act of feeding; it is a profound moment of connection. The baby's mouth envelops the breast, drawing the nipple deep into their mouth. A proper latch is not just about feeding; it's about ensuring the baby is comfortable and able to effectively extract milk. The initial latch sets the stage for a successful breastfeeding journey, shaping the baby's understanding of the breast and establishing the foundation for milk production.

II. Birth Interventions and Their Impact on the Golden Hour

A. Cesarean Sections: Adapting Skin-to-Skin Contact in Surgical Births

In the realm of cesarean sections, the Golden Hour takes on a unique form. While the immediate skin-to-skin contact may be challenged by the surgical environment, there are ways to adapt and ensure this precious connection is not lost. Gentle cesareans, also known as family-centered or natural cesareans, prioritize the emotional and physical well-being of both mother and baby.

During a gentle cesarean, the surgical drape is lowered, allowing the mother to witness the birth of her baby. As soon as the baby is born, they are placed on the mother's chest, facilitating skin-to-skin contact. Even in the midst of the sterile environment, the warmth of the mother's body and her reassuring touch provide the baby with a sense of security.

B. Inductions and Augmentations: Supporting Natural Rhythms

In cases where inductions or augmentations are necessary, preserving the integrity of the Golden Hour is paramount. The process of inducing or augmenting labor can sometimes lead to a cascade of interventions, potentially disrupting the natural flow of the Golden Hour. However, by approaching these interventions mindfully, the beauty of the Golden Hour can still be embraced.

Inductions, often initiated due to medical concerns or post-term pregnancies, can create challenges in the birthing process. However, even in induced labors, the birthing team can work collaboratively to create an environment conducive to skin-to-skin contact immediately after birth. Monitoring the baby's well-being continuously allows for adjustments in interventions, ensuring that the natural rhythm.

C. Medical Procedures and the Golden Hour

Amidst the medical assessments and procedures that often follow birth, it is essential to prioritize the uninterrupted bonding between mother and baby. While some assessments are necessary, especially in the case of medical complications, it is vital to create a balance between ensuring the baby's well-being and safeguarding the Golden Hour.

Routine newborn assessments, such as Apgar scoring and measurements, can be performed while the baby is on the mother's chest. This approach, known as "in-arms assessments," allows medical professionals to conduct necessary checks without separating the baby from the mother. By adopting this practice, the baby can remain in the comforting embrace of the Golden Hour, promoting a seamless transition into breastfeeding.

As we delve deeper into the intricacies of the Golden Hour, we uncover the delicate balance between the natural instincts of both mother and baby and the medical considerations that may arise. By understanding the physiological significance of this sacred time and embracing adaptable approaches to interventions, we can ensure that the Golden Hour serves as a foundation for a harmonious breastfeeding journey, setting the stage for a thriving mother-baby bond.

Chapter 3: Nurturing the First Latch

In the heart of the birthing room, where the echoes of the first cries blend with the mother's tender whispers, a dance begins – the dance of the first latch. In this chapter, we explore the intricate interplay of nature's design and the nurturing guidance of mothers. We unravel the physiological and emotional nuances of the first latch, honoring the instinctual wisdom of both mother and baby. Together, we embark on a journey that celebrates the art of breastfeeding, a dance that begins with the sacred rhythm of the first latch.

I. The Dance of Instinct: Understanding Baby's Cues

A. The Rooting Reflex: Nature's Compass

At the heart of the first latch lies the rooting reflex, a primal instinct that guides newborns toward their source of nourishment. With a gentle stroke on the cheek, the baby turns toward the sensation, mouth agape, seeking the comforting touch of the breast. This natural response, finely tuned by evolution, ensures that even in the dim light of the birthing room, the baby finds its way to the mother's breast, guided by the subtlest of cues.

B. Sensory Cues: The Language of Connection

The newborn arrives in the world equipped with finely tuned senses – a keen sense of smell, touch, and taste. The mother's unique scent, the warmth of her skin, and the taste of her milk form a sensory tapestry that lures the baby in, creating an irresistible path to the breast. In this dance of connection, the baby's senses align with the mother's, weaving a bond that transcends words.

C. The Latch Sequence: A Symphony of Nurturing Guidance

Within the first latch lies the essence of successful breastfeeding. A deep, comfortable latch is not just about feeding; it's about ensuring the baby can extract milk effectively while ensuring the mother's comfort. The latch sequence, beginning with the baby's wide-open mouth, the engulfing of the breast, and the rhythmic suckling, is a dance of mutual understanding. In this sequence, both mother and baby find their rhythm, orchestrating a symphony of nourishment and love.

II. Maternal Guidance and Support: Nurturing the Breastfeeding Connection

A. The Breastfeeding Position: Crafting a Comfortable Nest

Breastfeeding positions are more than just physical arrangements; they are nurturing environments where the baby feels safe and supported. The cradle hold, the football hold, and the laid-back breastfeeding position each offer unique advantages. Exploring these positions allows the mother to find the one that ensures both her comfort and the baby's ease of latching. The positioning of pillows and cushions acts as the foundation, creating a nest where the dance of breastfeeding can unfold harmoniously.

B. Breast Support: Cradling Comfort

In the dance of breastfeeding, proper breast support plays a pivotal role. Nursing pillows and cushions are not mere accessories; they are silent partners in the nurturing of the first latch. Supporting the breast ensures a comfortable angle for the baby, reducing strain on the mother's back and shoulders. In the gentle cradle of proper breast support, the baby finds a stable platform from which to dance into the world of nourishment.

C. Gentle Nudges and Encouragement: Guiding the Dance

Breastfeeding is an art, and like any art form, it thrives on guidance and encouragement. The art of gentle nudges involves subtle adjustments – a shift in the baby's position, a gentle nudge to deepen the latch, or a calming word of reassurance. In this dance, the mother is the guiding force, gently nudging the baby toward a deeper latch, ensuring optimal milk transfer and her own comfort. Encouragement is the melody of the dance, a soft hum that resonates with love and support, fostering a tranquil environment where both mother and baby can find their rhythm.

III. Overcoming Challenges with Patience and Persistence: Honoring the Dance

A. Latch Difficulties: A Compassionate Approach

Even in the most harmonious dances, challenges may arise. Latch difficulties, often a result of shallow latch or nipple pain, can disrupt the flow of the breastfeeding dance. A compassionate approach, marked by patience and persistence, becomes the guiding light. Addressing these challenges involves techniques such as the breast sandwich, nipple shields, and seeking professional guidance. The dance may falter, but with persistence and unwavering support, it finds its rhythm once more.

B. Engorgement and Flat Nipples: Embracing Variations

The dance of breastfeeding embraces the unique contours of every mother and baby. Engorgement and flat or inverted nipples are variations in the dance, not barriers. Engorgement, a natural part of the breastfeeding journey, can be managed with techniques such as warm compresses and gentle hand expression. Flat or invertednipples find their place in the dance with the use of breast shells, nipple shields, and gentle coaxing. In the embrace of acceptance and adaptability, the dance continues, honoring the individuality of every breastfeeding pair.

C. Nipple Shield Considerations: A Temporary Partner

For some mothers and babies, the dance may require the gentle presence of a nipple shield. A nipple shield, when used under professional guidance, becomes a temporary partner in the dance. It offers a bridge, guiding the baby toward a deeper latch and easing challenges such as latch difficulties and inverted nipples. With patience and proper usage, the nipple shield becomes a stepping stone, a companion on the journey toward a harmonious breastfeeding relationship.

In the dance of the first latch, we witness the exquisite harmony of nature and nurture. Guided by the baby's instinct and the mother's nurturing presence, the first latch becomes a testament to the profound connection between mother and child. With each subtle cue, each gentle adjustment, and each moment of patient persistence, the dance unfolds, laying the foundation for a joyful and nurturing breastfeeding journey. In the embrace of this dance, the mother and baby find not just nourishment, but a deep, enduring bond that becomes the heart of their breastfeeding relationship.

Chapter 4: Herbal Remedies and Natural Treatments for Breastfeeding Complications

In the lush gardens of nature, where healing blossoms and remedies are whispered on the wind, mothers find solace and support. In this chapter, we explore the age-old wisdom of herbal remedies and natural treatments, crafted by the Earth herself, to nurture breastfeeding mothers through challenges. These gentle allies, rooted in tradition and validated by modern knowledge, offer holistic solutions for common breastfeeding complications. With the touch of herbal wisdom, we embrace the healing power of nature, paving the way for a resilient and harmonious breastfeeding journey.

I. Herbal Allies: Nature's Gifts for Lactation

A. Fenugreek: The Milk-Eliciting Herb

Fenugreek, with its delicate leaves and aromatic seeds, stands as a symbol of abundant milk supply in herbal lore. This herb, rich in phytoestrogens, supports milk production by stimulating mammary glands. Learn how to prepare fenugreek tea, tinctures, or incorporate it into delicious lactation-enhancing recipes to naturally boost milk supply.

B. Blessed Thistle: Nature's Galactagogue

Embraced for centuries as a galactagogue, blessed thistle supports lactation by enhancing milk flow. Discover the art of crafting blessed thistle infusions and tinctures, and understand its gentle yet effective impact on milk production. Explore the soothing benefits of blessed thistle tea, providing comfort and nourishment to both body and soul.

C. Nettle: The Nutrient-Rich Nurturer

Nettle, with its vibrant green leaves, is a powerhouse of essential nutrients. Rich in vitamins and minerals, nettle tea becomes a nurturing elixir for breastfeeding mothers. Dive into the world of nettle infusions, exploring their role in replenishing vital nutrients, promoting overall well-being, and fortifying the milk supply.

D. Fennel: The Sweet Sip of Nourishment

Fennel, with its delicate fronds and aromatic seeds, emerges as a delightful addition to the breastfeeding journey. Revered for its ability to promote lactation, fennel tea becomes a cherished ritual for mothers seeking natural support. Explore the art of brewing fennel tea, infusing the air with its sweet aroma and instilling a sense of calm. Discover fennel-infused recipes, transforming simple meals into nourishing feasts that enhance milk production and nurture the breastfeeding bond.

E. Sunflower Lecithin: The Lactation Facilitator

Sunflower lecithin, derived from sunflower seeds, emerges as a valuable ally in addressing breastfeeding challenges. Known for its emulsifying properties, sunflower lecithin aids in preventing blocked ducts and promotes smooth milk flow. Learn the art of incorporating sunflower lecithin supplements into the daily routine, ensuring the gentle passage of milk, and nurturing breast health. In the subtle presence of sunflower lecithin, mothers find reassurance, allowing the dance of breastfeeding to flow with ease.

II. Addressing Common Concerns: Herbal Solutions for Breastfeeding Challenges

A. Mastitis: Herbal Soothing and Immune Support

Mastitis, a painful inflammation of the breast tissue, finds its match in herbal remedies. Discover the antimicrobial properties of echinacea and the soothing qualities of calendula. Learn to craft poultices, compresses, and herbal salves that alleviate pain, reduce inflammation, and support the body's natural healing process.

B. Thrush: Herbal Antifungal Allies

Thrush, a stubborn fungal infection, requires delicate yet effective remedies. Explore the antifungal properties of garlic, gentian violet, and grapefruit seed extract. Delve into the world of probiotic-rich foods and herbal infusions that restore balance to the body, promoting a healthy breastfeeding experience.

C. Blocked Ducts: Herbal Unblockers and Massage Oils

Blocked ducts, a common challenge for breastfeeding mothers, can be gently eased with the aid of herbal allies. Learn the art of creating herbal massage oils infused with lavender, chamomile, and cypress, soothing both physical discomfort and emotional tension. Herbal compresses, warm and fragrant, become tender companions in resolving blocked ducts, restoring the free flow of milk.

III. Healing with Herbs: Soothing Sore Nipples and Promoting Healing

A. Calendula: The Petal-Soft Healer

Calendula, with its golden petals, embodies healing and regeneration. Explore the art of creating calendula-infused oils and salves, providing a protective shield for sore nipples. Dive into the world of herbal sitz baths, where the soothing embrace of calendula promotes healing and relaxation, nurturing both body and spirit.

B. Comfrey: Nature's Knitting Herb

Comfrey, revered for its tissue-repairing properties, becomes a powerful ally for healing cracked nipples. Discover the art of creating comfrey poultices and ointments, gently encouraging the skin to mend. Learn to embrace the herbal wisdom of comfrey-infused oils, fostering a nurturing environment for healing and renewal.

C. Lavender: The Fragrant Soother

Lavender, with its calming aroma, brings tranquility to both body and mind. Explore the world of lavender-infused creams and balms, offering relief to sore and cracked nipples. Discover the therapeutic benefits of lavender essential oil, transforming simple massage oils into soothing elixirs that promote relaxation and healing.

In the gentle embrace of herbal remedies, breastfeeding mothers find not just physical relief, but also emotional nourishment. These natural solutions, rooted in the Earth's wisdom, become companions on the breastfeeding journey, offering comfort, healing, and the reassurance that nature herself is a steadfast ally. With the touch of herbal grace, mothers are empowered to navigate challenges with resilience, embracing the healing power of the

Earth as they nurture both their babies and their own well-being.

Chapter 5: PUMPING

In the rhythmic hum of the breast pump, mothers discover a modern-day companion in their breastfeeding journey. Pumping, often seen as a practical necessity, transcends the mechanical process; it becomes an art, a dance of dedication, and a profound expression of love. In this chapter, we delve into the art of pumping, exploring techniques, tools, and tender moments that transform this act into a nurturing ritual. From choosing the right pump to mastering the art of expressing milk, pumping becomes not just a means to provide nourishment but an intimate extension of the breastfeeding bond.

I. Choosing the Perfect Pump: A Mother's Muse

A. Manual vs. Electric Pumps: Finding Your Rhythm

Dive into the world of breast pumps, understanding the nuances of manual and electric options. Manual pumps, with their simplicity and portability, offer a hands-on approach, allowing mothers to control the rhythm and pressure. Electric pumps, with their efficiency and convenience, provide a powerful yet gentle suction, mimicking the natural breastfeeding pattern. Explore the advantages of each, helping mothers find the pump that aligns with their lifestyle, needs, and comfort.

B. Pumping Accessories: Tools of the Trade

Explore the realm of pumping accessories, from breast shields and flanges to storage bags and cooling packs. Understand the significance of correct sizing, ensuring comfort and optimal milk extraction. Dive into the art of hands-free pumping, embracing bra inserts and pumping bras that allow mothers to multitask while nurturing their milk supply. In the world of pumping accessories, mothers find the support they need, transforming pumping into a seamless and comfortable experience.

II. Mastering the Art of Pumping: Techniques and Tips

A. Pumping Rhythms: Embracing the Natural Flow

Delve into the art of pumping rhythms, discovering the natural ebb and flow of milk production. Learn techniques to initiate letdown, including visualizing the baby, using scents, or gentle breast massage. Understand the importance of relaxation and comfort, creating a serene environment that promotes the free flow of milk. Explore the concept of hands-on pumping, employing breast compressions and massage to maximize milk output. In the dance of pumping rhythms, mothers find harmony, allowing milk to flow effortlessly.

B. Pumping Schedules: Balancing Supply and Demand

Unlock the secrets of pumping schedules, finding the delicate balance between supply and demand. Explore pumping frequency, understanding how often to pump to maintain milk supply and meet the baby's needs. Dive into the world of power pumping, a technique that mimics cluster feeding, encouraging the body to produce more milk. Embrace the concept of dream pumping, utilizing nighttime hours to express milk, promoting relaxation and enhancing milk production. In the realm of pumping schedules, mothers discover a tailored approach that ensures a thriving milk supply while honoring their unique breastfeeding journey.

III. Storage and Handling: Preserving Liquid Gold

Navigate the intricacies of breast milk storage and handling, preserving the precious liquid gold that mothers work so diligently to express. Explore proper storage temperatures and durations, ensuring the safety and nutritional value of stored breast milk. Understand the significance of labeling and organizing stored milk, optimizing freshness and convenience. Delve into the world of milk thawing and warming techniques, maintaining the integrity of breast milk while preparing it for the baby's nourishment. In the art of storage and handling, mothers find confidence, knowing that their expressed milk is preserved with care and dedication.

IV. Nurturing the Bond: Incorporating Pumped Milk into the Breastfeeding Relationship

Pumping, while practical, becomes a deeply emotional act when infused with intention and connection. Explore the art of introducing pumped milk to the baby, whether through bottle feeding or alternative feeding methods. Embrace paced bottle feeding, a technique that promotes a natural suck-swallow-breathe rhythm, ensuring the baby's comfort and reducing nipple confusion. Discover the significance of skin-to-skin contact during bottle feeding, preserving the emotional bond between mother and baby. In the nurturing embrace of pumped milk, mothers find the freedom to share the feeding experience while preserving the breastfeeding relationship.

V. Pumping Challenges and Solutions: Overcoming Hurdles with Grace

Acknowledge the challenges that can arise in the pumping journey, from low milk output to discomfort and time constraints. Explore troubleshooting techniques, understanding the role of proper flange fit, pump settings, and relaxation techniques in overcoming pumping hurdles. Delve into the emotional aspects of pumping, offering guidance on managing stress, self-care, and seeking support. Embrace the concept of milk supply fluctuations, understanding the natural rhythm of breastfeeding, and adapting pumping techniques accordingly. In the face of challenges, mothers find resilience, navigating the pumping journey with grace and determination.

In the art of pumping, mothers discover not

just a practical necessity but a profound expression of love and dedication. With each rhythmic pulse of the pump, they nurture their milk supply and the breastfeeding bond, infusing the act with intention, connection, and unwavering love. Pumping becomes not just a means to provide nourishment but a testament to the mother's commitment, transforming a mechanical process into a deeply meaningful ritual. In the gentle cadence of the breast pump, mothers find the melody of their breastfeeding journey, creating harmonious notes that resonate with love, dedication, and the enduring bond between mother and child.

Chapter 6: Weaning with Love

In the twilight of breastfeeding, as the baby grows and the nursing relationship evolves, mothers embark on a tender journey – the art of weaning. Weaning, often seen as a milestone, transcends the physical act of breastfeeding; it becomes a profound emotional transition for both mother and child. In this chapter, we explore the delicate art of weaning, embracing the process with love and grace. From gentle approaches to understanding emotional nuances, we navigate the path of weaning, honoring the sacred bond while allowing both mother and child to embrace new beginnings.

I. Embracing Gentle Weaning: A Slow Unraveling

A. Child-Led Weaning: Honoring Natural Timing

Child-led weaning, guided by the child's readiness and cues, becomes a gentle approach to the weaning journey. Explore the signs of a child's readiness to wean, from decreased interest in breastfeeding to embracing solid foods with enthusiasm. Understand the importance of emotional readiness, allowing the child to navigate the transition at their own pace. Embrace the concept of gradual weaning, offering comfort and support as the child naturally reduces nursing sessions. In child-led weaning, mothers find the beauty of allowing the process to unfold with patience and respect.

B. Mother-Led Weaning: Nurturing Transition with Compassion

Mother-led weaning, driven by the mother's intuition and considerations, becomes another pathway in the weaning journey. Explore the reasons for mother-led weaning, whether due to medical concerns, emotional readiness, or the mother's personal boundaries. Understand the importance of clear communication and consistency, ensuring that the child feels secure and supported throughout the transition. Embrace the power of comfort items and alternative soothing techniques, offering solace and reassurance to the child during the weaning process. In mother-led weaning, mothers find the strength to navigate the transition with love and compassion.

II. The Emotional Landscape of Weaning: Nurturing Heart and Soul

A. Navigating Emotional Challenges: Tears, Comfort, and Connection

Acknowledge the emotional challenges that can arise during weaning, both for the child and the mother. Explore the concept of nursing ceremonies, allowing the child to say goodbye to breastfeeding in a meaningful way. Delve into the world of comfort items, embracing transitional objects that offer solace and security. Understand the significance of extra cuddles, gentle words, and unlimited love, nurturing the emotional connection during the weaning process. In the midst of tears and comfort, mothers find the strength to navigate the emotional landscape, offering understanding, reassurance, and unwavering love.

B. Embracing the New Normal: Rituals and Transitions

Embrace the concept of rituals and transitions, allowing the weaning process to unfold within the framework of meaningful ceremonies. Explore the art of creating weaning rituals, whether through special songs, stories, or keepsakes that celebrate the breastfeeding journey. Understand the importance of gentle transitions, offering new soothing techniques and bonding activities that replace breastfeeding. Dive into the world of open communication, ensuring that the child feels heard, understood, and valued throughout the weaning process. In the embrace of rituals and transitions, mothers and children find the strength to move forward, embracing the new normal with love, grace, and a deep sense of connection.

III. Nurturing the Mother's Well-Being: Self-Care and Reflection

Acknowledge the impact of weaning on the mother's emotional well-being, understanding that this transition is a significant moment in her motherhood journey. Explore the concept of self-care, encouraging mothers to engage in activities that bring them joy, relaxation, and a sense of fulfillment. Delve into the world of reflection, allowing mothers to honor the breastfeeding journey, celebrating the moments of connection, love, and nurturing. Understand the importance of seeking support, whether through friends, family, or professional counselors, as mothers navigate the emotional complexities of weaning. In the embrace of self-care and reflection, mothers find the space to honor their emotions, allowing the weaning journey to unfold with grace and self-compassion.

In the delicate tapestry of weaning, mothers and children find the threads of love, understanding, and resilience. Weaning becomes not just a physical transition but a profound emotional journey, marked by the nurturing embrace of love and grace. With each step, mothers and children navigate the path together, finding solace in one another's arms, and embracing the new chapter with a heart full of gratitude, love, and the enduring bond of motherhood.

Chapter 7: The Sanctuary of Support

Motherhood, a journey both beautiful and challenging, is a sacred endeavor that flourishes within the embrace of a supportive community. This chapter delves into the profound impact of these communities, exploring the powerful connections that nurture mothers with understanding, encouragement, and love. From partners and friends to healthcare providers and online networks, the sanctuary of support becomes a haven where mothers find solace, share their triumphs and tribulations, and discover the strength of collective nurturing.

I. Partners: Pillars of Strength and

Encouragement

Partners, the unwavering pillars of a mother's world, play a pivotal role in her journey. Explore the significance of emotional support, where partners provide a safe space for mothers to express their fears, dreams, and challenges. Understand the importance of shared responsibilities, allowing partners to actively participate in childcare and household tasks, providing mothers the gift of time and rest. Delve into the realm of shared decision-making, where partners and mothers collaboratively navigate the parenting landscape, fostering unity and mutual respect. In the steadfast presence of partners, mothers find the courage to face the complexities of parenthood with resilience and grace.

II. Friends and Family: The Tapestry of Unconditional Love

Friends and family, the threads of unconditional love, weave a tapestry of emotional connection around mothers. Explore the significance of empathetic listening, where loved ones provide a compassionate ear, allowing mothers to share their thoughts and feelings without judgment. Understand the importance of practical support, as friends and family assist with childcare, household chores, and meal preparation, easing the burdens of daily responsibilities. Delve into the world of shared celebrations, where friends and family acknowledge mothers' achievements, creating a sense of pride and belonging. In the embrace of friends and family, mothers find the reassurance that they are cherished and supported, allowing them to navigate motherhood with confidence and joy.

III. Healthcare Providers: Guardians of Maternal Well-being

Healthcare providers, the guardians of maternal health, offer expert guidance and compassionate care to mothers. Explore the significance of respectful prenatal care, where healthcare providers empower mothers with knowledge, ensuring a healthy and supported pregnancy. Understand the importance of personalized birthing experiences, where providers respect mothers' choices, creating a positive and empowering birthing environment. Delve into the realm of postpartum support, where healthcare professionals offer guidance on breastfeeding, emotional well-being, and newborn care, nurturing mothers through the early days of motherhood. In the expertise and compassion of healthcare providers, mothers find the guidance and reassurance they need to navigate the complexities of motherhood with confidence and trust.

IV. Online Communities and Support Groups: Virtual Empathy and Connection

Online communities and support groups, the digital threads of connection, offer mothers a virtual sanctuary where they can share experiences, seek advice, and offer support to others. Explore the significance of online forums and social media groups, where mothers find empathy and understanding from those facing similar challenges. Understand the power of shared narratives, where stories inspire and reassure others, fostering a sense of community and belonging. Delve into the world of virtual resources, where online platforms provide access to expert advice, parenting resources, and emotional support, enriching mothers' knowledge and confidence. In the virtual empathy and connection of online communities, mothers find a diverse and inclusive circle of support, expanding their perspectives and nurturing their sense of community.

V. Advocacy and Community Initiatives: Fostering a Supportive Society

Advocacy and community initiatives, the driving forces of social change, play a vital role in nurturing mothers and families. Explore the significance of breastfeeding-friendly spaces and workplace policies, where mothers are supported, fostering acceptance and normalcy. Understand the importance of mental health awareness campaigns, offering education and resources to support emotional well-being, breaking the stigma surrounding mental health challenges. Delve into the world of parental leave policies and family support programs, where parents receive the time and resources needed to nurture their families without sacrificing financial stability. In the advocacy and community initiatives, mothers find a supportive society that values their well-being and recognizes their contributions, nurturing them to thrive as mothers and individuals.

In the sanctuary of support, mothers find the nurturing embrace of understanding, empathy, and love. It is within this sanctuary that they draw strength, wisdom, and resilience, allowing them to navigate the challenges of motherhood with grace and confidence. From partners and friends to healthcare providers and online communities, each thread of connection enriches the tapestry of motherhood, creating a supportive environment where mothers can blossom, nurture their families, and embrace the journey of parenthood with boundless love and endless gratitude

Motherhood, a sacred journey of love and nurturing, is not undertaken in isolation. It flourishes within a circle of support, where mothers find strength, wisdom, and reassurance. This chapter delves into the profound impact of supportive communities, exploring the web of connections that cradle mothers with understanding, encouragement, and love. From partners and friends to healthcare providers and online communities, the circle of support becomes a sanctuary where mothers find solace, share their joys and challenges, and discover the power of collective nurturing.

I. The Role of Partners: Unwavering Pillars of Support

Partners, the steadfast companions on the journey of parenthood, play a pivotal role in nurturing mothers. Explore the significance of emotional support, where partners provide a safe space for mothers to express their feelings, fears, and triumphs. Understand the importance of shared responsibilities, where partners actively participate in childcare, allowing mothers moments of rest and self-care. Delve into the world of shared decision-making, where partners and mothers collaborate in parenting choices, creating a harmonious and united front. In the unwavering support of partners, mothers find the strength to embrace the challenges of parenthood with grace and resilience.

II. Friends and Family: The Tapestry of Emotional Connection

Friends and family, the threads of emotional connection, weave a tapestry of love and understanding around mothers. Explore the significance of empathetic listening, where friends and family members lend a compassionate ear, offering mothers a space to share their thoughts and feelings. Understand the importance of practical support, where loved ones assist with household tasks, childcare, and meal preparation, alleviating the burdens of daily responsibilities. Delve into the world of celebratory moments, where friends and family acknowledge mothers' achievements, both big and small, fostering a sense of pride and accomplishment. In the embrace of friends and family, mothers find the reassurance that they are cherished and supported, allowing them to navigate motherhood with confidence and joy.

III. Healthcare Providers: Guiding with Expertise and Compassion

Maternal healthcare providers, often seen as the guardians of maternal and infant health, offer expert guidance and compassionate care to mothers. Explore the significance of respectful and informed prenatal care, where healthcare providers empower mothers with knowledge, ensuring a healthy and supported pregnancy. Understand the importance of personalized birthing experiences, where healthcare providers respect mothers' birth preferences, creating a positive and empowering birthing environment. Delve into the world of postpartum support, where healthcare professionals offer guidance on breastfeeding, emotional well-being, and newborn care, nurturing mothers through the early days of motherhood. In the expertise and compassion of the correct healthcare provider, mothers find the guidance and reassurance they need to navigate the complexities of motherhood with confidence and trust.

IV. Online Communities and Support Groups: Virtual Empathy and Connection

Online communities and support groups, the digital threads of connection, offer mothers a virtual sanctuary where they can share their experiences, seek advice, and offer support to others. Explore the significance of online forums and social media groups, where mothers find empathy and understanding from individuals facing similar challenges. Understand the power of shared narratives, where mothers' stories inspire and reassure others, fostering a sense of community and belonging. Delve into the world of virtual resources, where online platforms provide access to expert advice, parenting resources, and emotional support, enriching mothers' knowledge and confidence. In the virtual empathy and connection of online communities, mothers find a diverse and inclusive circle of support, expanding their perspectives and nurturing their sense of community.

V. Advocacy and Community Initiatives: Fostering a Supportive Society

Advocacy and community initiatives, the driving forces of social change, play a vital role in nurturing mothers and families. Explore the significance of breastfeeding-friendly initiatives in public spaces and workplaces, where mothers are supported in their breastfeeding journey, fostering a sense of acceptance and normalcy. Understand the importance of mental health awareness campaigns, where mothers receive education and resources to support their emotional well-being, breaking the stigma surrounding mental health challenges. Delve into the world of parental leave policies and family support programs, where parents are granted the time and resources to nurture their families without sacrificing their financial stability. In the advocacy and community initiatives, mothers find a supportive society that values their well-being and recognizes their contributions, nurturing them to thrive as mothers and individuals.

In the circle of support, mothers find the nurturing embrace of understanding, empathy, and love. It is within this circle that they draw strength, wisdom, and resilience, allowing them to navigate the challenges of motherhood with grace and confidence. From partners and friends to healthcare providers and online communities, each thread of connection enriches the tapestry of motherhood, creating a supportive environment where mothers can blossom, nurture their families, and embrace the journey of parenthood with boundless love and endless gratitude.

ABOUT THE AUTHOR

In the beautiful Grande Ronde Valley of eastern corner of Oregon, I find my purpose as a mother, doula, educator, herbalist, holistic health coach, and storyteller. Living on our farm, surrounded by the comfort of chickens, the laughter of my family, and the loyalty of our dogs, I have discovered part of my purpose on this earth is working to better our world's maternal health outcomes.

As a doula, I stand beside mothers, guiding them with unwavering support through the sacred passage of birth. In my role as a breastfeeding educator, I empower mothers with knowledge, remedies and the art of breastfeeding, helping them find confidence in their journey. As an herbalist, I craft remedies from nature's bounty, offering healing and comfort to those in need. My life is a testament to my advocacy for maternal health, my dedication to holistic well-being, educating the masses, and my profound love for the art of motherhood. Each day, I find fulfillment in guiding my community, empowering mothers, and healing myself in the process. My story is one of resilience, compassion, and boundless love, woven into the tapestry of life in the heart of Oregon.

Elisha Anderson

Made in the USA
Las Vegas, NV
14 October 2023

79079088R00036